SDI SCUBA DIVING INTERNATIONAL TECHNICAL DIVING INTERNATIONAL TDI

CPROX1st and AED

The common sense lifesaving program

by Warren Smith MD

Scuba Diving International® / Technical Diving International®

Credits

CPROX1st and AED - The common sense lifesaving program
Publisher:
International Training
Phone: 888-778-9073 Fax: 877-436-7096
www.tdisdi.com email: worldhq@tdisdi.com

Executive Editor Brian Carney
Editor Steve Lewis
Author: Warren L. Smith MD
Art Director: Lynn Hendrickson

Photography / Illustrations:
Doug Arnberg (www.exploreH2O.com)
Harry Averill
Bret Gilliam
Warren Smith MD

Reviewers and Contributors:
Donna Bissett
Sean Harrison
Paul Montgomery

Disclaimer:
All diving activities have inherent risks involved. Each individual diver engaging in any form of diving must accept the risks and **accept** responsibility for their own actions. The author and publisher assume no liability to anyone for loss, damage, injury or death caused by any error or omission in the work. Any and all such liability is disclaimed. The information in this manual pertains to CPROX1st, and is only to be used as a supplement to recognized training by a certified SDI CPROX1st Instructor. This manual cannot replace professional instruction and good judgment.

ISBN: 1-931451-39-7 **Product ID #: 410024**

Table of Contents

Common Sense Lifesaving

What Is Common Sense Lifesaving?

Welcome to Common Sense Lifesaving. This course will forever change the way you respond to emergencies. It has been developed from the ground up to integrate the four most important lifesaving skill sets into one fun, practical, and easy to remember course. Common Sense Lifesaving is intended to provide potential rescuers, regardless of background, with an intuitive, common sense approach to helping the victim(s) of an emergency.

Why Common Sense Lifesaving?

Traditional medical education including most CPR and first aid courses are "diagnosis centered." They attempt to encompass basic anatomy, relevant physiology and dozens of different diseases and injuries. They require you to memorize the ideal set of actions and treatments for each of many possible circumstances. Finally, you are expected to remember and apply all this information in an actual emergency.

You are asked to commit time and resources to different courses on different days in an attempt to cover all of the topics. Even if you are able to remain focused throughout these sessions, it is unlikely you will be able to assimilate all of the information and apply it in an emergency months or years later. In fact, it has been observed that in actual emergencies where CPR would have been beneficial, trained bystanders have failed to act because, "I couldn't remember what I was supposed to do," or "I was afraid I would hurt (the victim)" (JAMA 1992, vol. 268, no. 16).

It is apparent that for a lifesaving course to be truly effective, you must not only be presented accurate and useful information, you must be able to remember and apply that training in an actual emergency – long after you have completed the course. Then, you need the confidence to act without fear of harming the victim or being subjected to legal action.

How Common Sense Lifesaving Works

Common Sense Lifesaving is condition-centered. That is, instead of focusing on the anatomy, physiology and diagnosis of an injury or illness and then applying medical algorithms, Common Sense Lifesaving simply observes the condition (ex. bleeding) and applies the intuitive response (ex. pressure) to it. Using Common Sense Lifesaving doesn't require any medical knowledge, rescuers simply respond to the physical condition they are presented with. For example, we instinctively respond to "hot" by applying cold, so we respond to a burn by cooling it. Instead, Common Sense Lifesaving reinforces this instinctive response to burns and encourages student's confidence to use it.

The same instinctive condition-response applies to the other categories of observed injuries; bleeding? - apply pressure, broken bone? - immobilize it, and so on. The condition-response approach to first-aid allows us to condense dozens of different disease and injury processes into just a few observable conditions. In fact, nearly every situation, for which first-aid or CPR is likely to be useful, can be categorized into one of just six observable conditions - the "6 Bs". These six Bs or basic conditions of emergency care are; Breathing, Bleeding, Broken, Burns, Bites and Baffled!

You won't have to memorize the 6 Bs. The only thing you need to remember is the correct response for each of the Bs. As you gain experience applying the 6 Bs in Common Sense Lifesaving, you will see the intuitive logic of each response.

What About Liability?

CPR and first-aid are stop gap skills provided to a person in need because more advanced care is not available. Doing anything reasonable to help a sick or injured person until they can get definitive medical help is generally better than doing nothing at all. As long as the rescuer uses common sense and acts in good faith, there is virtually no risk to either himself or the victim.

There are two reasonable questions to ask yourself about offering help to a sick or injured person.

1. What if I hurt the victim? By exercising common sense and following the simple, conditioned response guidelines of Common Sense Lifesaving, it is extremely unlikely that you will inflict further harm on a victim and very likely that you will be of some assistance.

2. Will I be held legally liable for a less than ideal outcome if I offer to help in an emergency. The answer is no, Good Samaritan Laws protect well-meaning rescuers from liability and are recognized throughout most of the world. There is no legal precedent for suing a rescuer who has acted in good faith?

Lifesaving Equipment Utilized or Recommended in Common Sense Lifesaving

- **This Student Manual**

- **Student Slate**
  The student manual in Common Sense Lifesaving has been summarized in a slate. You should keep your Common Sense Lifesaving slate in a convenient place in your everyday surroundings. This helps assure that important reference materials will be quickly accessible in an emergency!

- **Barrier Devices**
  You should always use protective gloves if they are available in an emergency. Barrier devices for CPR breathing are part of many emergency kits and are available for purchase.

- **Oro-nasal Mask**
  You should have the use of an oro-nasal mask when learning Common Sense Lifesaving. You are encouraged to purchase an oro-nasal mask of your own and keep it in a handy place (boat, RV, kitchen) for emergencies.

- **Old Clothing**
  Old clothes or towels are handy for demonstrating and practicing pressure and immobilization responses. They can also be used as barrier devices. Common Sense Lifesaving encourages learning using everyday items for lifesaving since they are often all that will be available in an actual emergency.

- **Makeshift Splint Materials**
  Practice with newspapers, a cardboard box or other locally available items that might be utilized to make splints.

- **Water**
  Water should be available from any safe source in the natural surroundings.

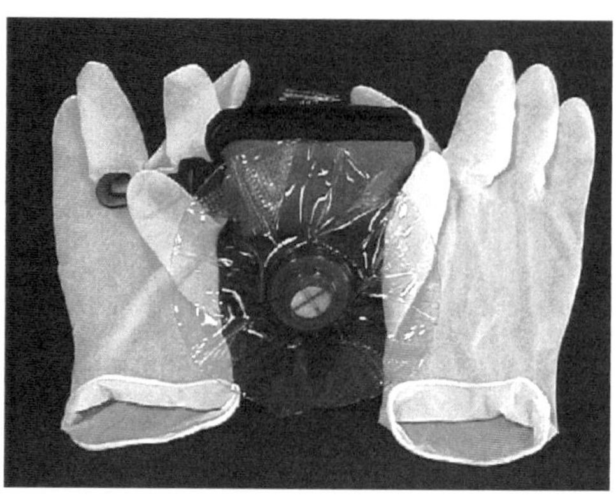

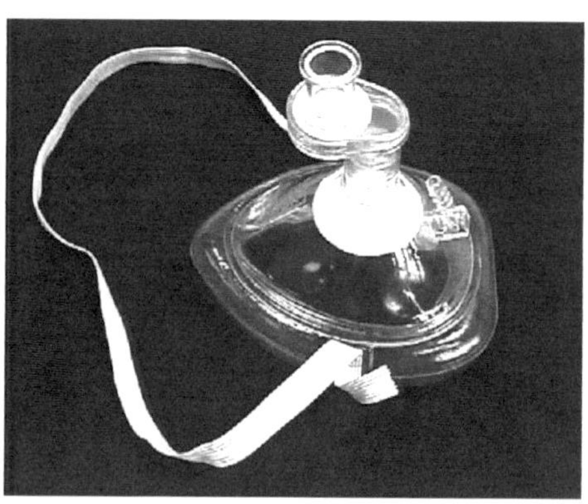

- **Oxygen**
  O2 bottle including delivery method, preferably non-rebreather mask and demand type valve with a face-mask if you intend to learn O2 administration.

- **Automatic External Defibrillator**
  An AED unit should be available for demonstration purposes.

Common Sense Lifesaving Course Outline

- **Body Structure and Function**
- **The 6 Basics**
- **"Other conditions"**
- **Giving O2 in the first aid setting**
- **CPR (O2)**
- **Use of the AED when available**
- **Transport of the sick and injured**
- **Instructor demonstration of approach and application**

Body Structure and Function

Lets start with simple review of human body parts and what they do, their "structure and function".

Figure 1-Blood flows in blood vessels from the heart through the lungs and to the rest of the body then flows back to the heart again. This process is called our circulation.

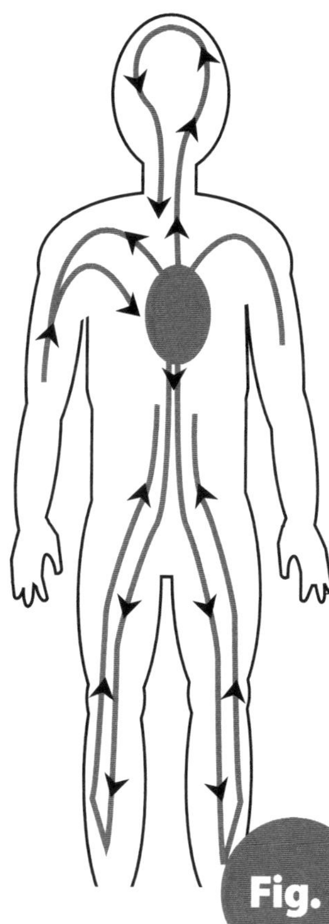

Fig. 1

Figure 2-Our two lungs take in air to provide oxygen to the circulation and remove carbon dioxide (CO_2) from the circulation. We breath in air to get oxygen into our lungs and we exhale air to get the CO_2 out of our lungs.

Figure 3-Our brain is in our skull and the spinal cord comes out of the bottom of it and passes down through our backbone. The spinal cord gives off nerves along its length that go to our arms, legs and all of our body parts. This lets our brain provide feeling and control to our body parts.

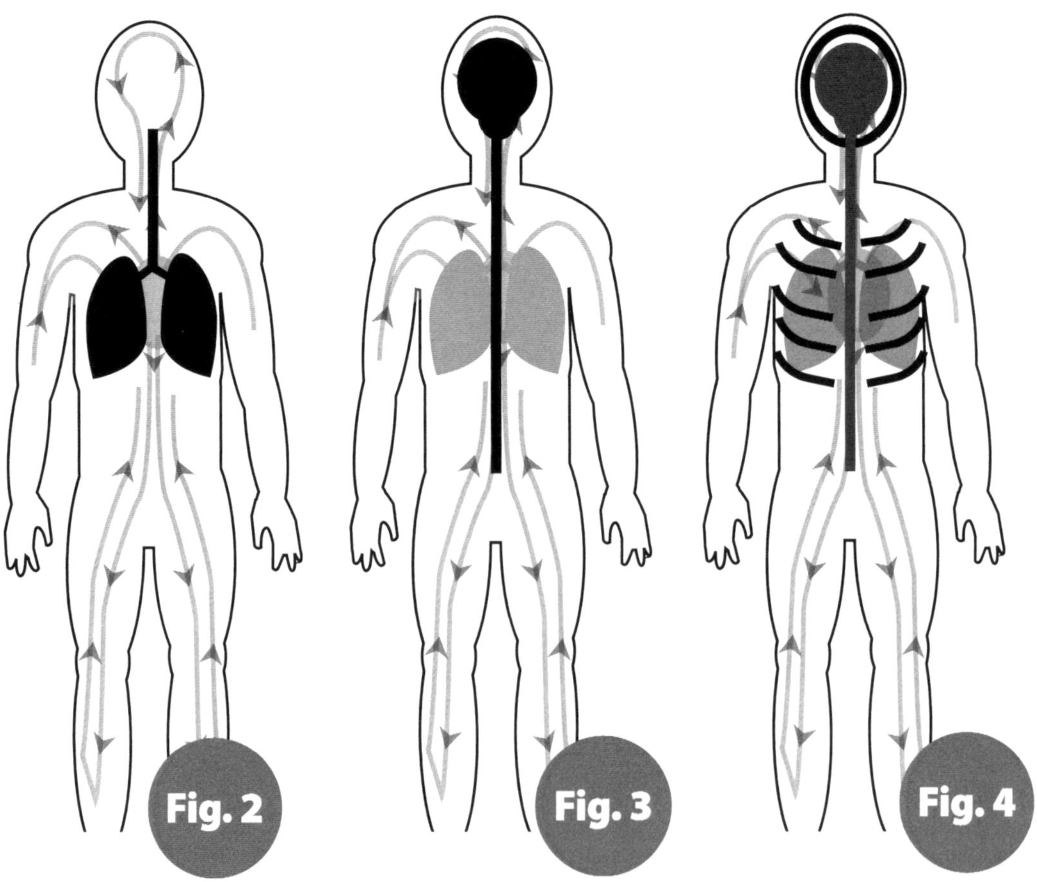

Figure 4-The skull protects our brain. Our ribs protect our lungs and upper abdominal organs. Our organs are soft and can be injured without it being apparent on the outside of our body.

The 6 Basics™ of First Aid

There is an almost infinite number of ways for people to become sick or injured. In Common Sense Lifesaving you will learn a very simple approach to first aid that will work in almost any situation.

The first-aid treatable aspects of almost every illness or injury fall into one of six basic observable conditions. Each of the six conditions begins with the letter "B" and just about all of the possibilities in each of the 6 Basic groups can be treated with the same response.

Breathing (absent) ➜ CPR

Breathing is absolutely essential to sustain life. Because a non-breathing victim will quickly die, the first condition to look for is the absence of a reasonably normal pattern of breathing. A "reasonably normal pattern of breathing" means someone who is breathing steadily and once every few seconds. To be satisfactory, a victim's breathing pattern should "make sense". For example, it makes sense that an anxious victim may be "hyperventilating" or a physically exhausted victim may be breathing deeply and rapidly. However, erratic, labored or gasping breathing, especially in an unconscious victim, may signal the need for CPR.

Common Sense Lifesaving will teach you a very easy to remember method of CPR, but first, let's review a very important maneuver that may help a choking victim and avoid the need for CPR altogether.

The Heimlich Maneuver

A victim who is believed to be choking on food or other matter may be breathing, but with great distress. A successful Heimlich maneuver may avert the need for CPR. The risk of harming a choking victim with this maneuver is minimal compared to the benefit of clearing their airway.

Although the Heimlich maneuver is normally taught in the standing or sitting position, if a choking victim has already fallen to the ground, he can be rolled to his back and several abdominal thrusts can be delivered from a position above the victim.

Even when the Heimlich maneuver is successful and a previously choking victim is breathing comfortably, you must watch them carefully for possible recurrent choking or inhalation of the foreign body that caused the choking episode. It is recommended that a victim of severe choking follow up with medical personnel as soon as possible. Remember, a choking victim that does not resume a satisfactory respiratory pattern may still require CPR.

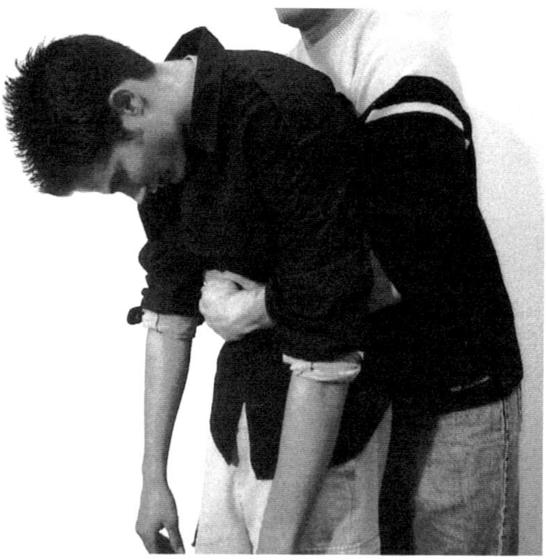

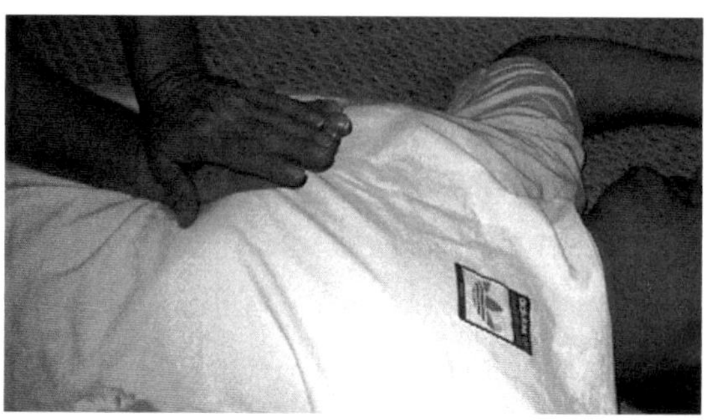

Using the abdominal thrust to clear an airway obstruction.

Bleeding → Pressure

Bleeding can occur with any injury. If bleeding is very minor and associated with a superficial wound, it may be possible to ignore it altogether. On the other hand, if the bleeding appears to be severe and continuous, it must be stopped before the blood supply reaches a critically low level in the body. Bleeding is the equivalent of a "leak" in the vascular system and the instinctive response to any leak is to apply pressure over the leak. Therefore the condition-response for bleeding is pressure. By applying pressure to reduce the blood flow, the body's powerful clotting mechanisms are given the opportunity to take over and help stop the bleeding.

Accidents and emergencies seldom occur under ideal circumstances.

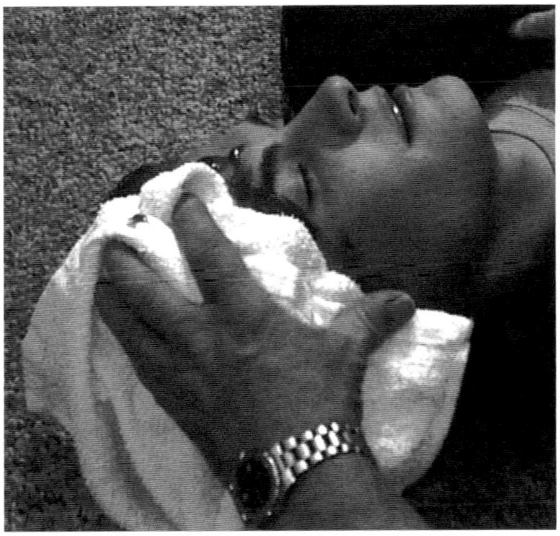

Using a Folded Towel as a Pressure Dressing

If there's a first-aid kit with sterile dressings at the scene of a bleeding emergency, it should be used. However, it is safe to assume that in the majority of bleeding emergencies, a supply of sterile wound dressings will not be available. Therefore, it is important to use the materials you have at hand.

There is minimal risk of causing infection by using everyday items to apply pressure to a bleeding wound. A reasonably clean article of clothing or a towel or blanket is nearly always available and can safely be used. These items are usually relatively free of dangerous germs. Additionally, a bleeding wound will tend to flush contaminants away. If infection does occur, it usually takes time to develop and can be addressed once the victim is under regular medical care. Therefore, the risk of infection is far outweighed by the benefit of stopping serious bleeding.

The amount of pressure you should apply is dependent on the amount of bleeding present. The goal is to slow the majority of blood loss over most of the bleeding area. It is extremely unlikely that the application of direct pressure will further injure a bleeding wound, so apply enough pressure to make the bleeding slow or stop.

The risk of exposure to blood products has been well publicized. Diseases like hepatitis and AIDS may be present in the blood of infected persons. For you to become infected, the victim's blood or body fluids must enter your circulation through a break in your skin. This means you would have to get a sufficient amount of blood or body fluids from an actively infected person into an open wound or crack in your skin. Even then, it is unlikely that you would develop an infection. Even direct needle sticks from infected patients into medical personnel seldom result in infection. So the chance of getting a dangerous infection from a bleeding victim is very, very small. Nevertheless, you should try to wear rubber gloves or keep a generous layer of material between you and a bleeding person's blood. As soon as you are finished assisting a bleeding victim, wash your hands and any other contact areas.

Broken → Immobilize

The next Basic is "broken", which most obviously refers to broken bones. If there is an obvious deformity of a person's body, especially around the extremities, further internal injuries can occur by the broken portion being moved. Therefore, the conditioned response to broken is immobilization; to prevent the fracture from being moved.

The most basic form of immobilization is simply to instruct the victim not to move the affected area. However, this is not always practical and some form of mechanical immobilization is often necessary. A professional grade splint is not likely to be immediately available in an emergency involving a broken bone. As in the case with other types of emergencies, using readily available materials is often the best alternative available to you.

If the victim has a possible neck or spine injury (any blow to the head, neck or body of a victim,) it is best to avoid moving him/her. When possible, the victim's neck should be immobilized as-is with a soft but firm support, like "sandbags", on either side. If the victim's head must be moved, for example to provide CPR or to move the victim to a safer location, then move it as slowly and as little as possible. If the victim is responsive, talk to him/her during the movement and ask him/her to tell you if there is any change in body sensation during the move. If possible, have a second rescuer stabilize the victim's head position during movement.

A broken neck is the most infamous and potentially destructive broken bone. First responders who suspect a broken neck may be reluctant to provide help to an injured victim for fear of inflicting spinal cord damage resulting in paralysis. Do not overemphasize these dangers. Remember that the first priority - even more important than protecting a possible spinal injury - is to restore breathing if necessary.

Fractures of the extremities are also treated with immobilization. Use rolled newspaper, folded cardboard or other available materials to demonstrate methods of splinting fractures, or suspected fractures of the extremities. Rope, belts, tape and other

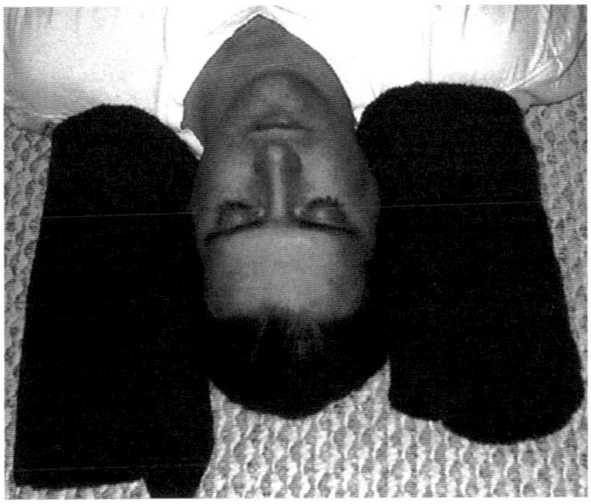

Head and neck "sandbagged" with two beach towels

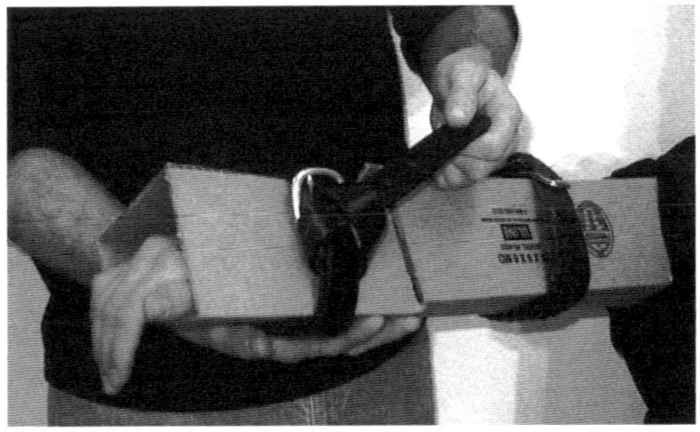

Makeshift Cardboard Splint

materials can be used to hold the splints in place. You should not attempt to "set" broken bones as "setting" requires blindly moving the ends of the broken bones, thus risking further internal injury. On the other hand, there is seldom any danger to immobilizing broken bones where they are while waiting for medical assistance.

When splinting an extremity, the goal is to extend the splint beyond the joints on either side of the area to be immobilized, if possible. For example, the splint on a broken forearm or wrist should include the elbow and hand.

Broken bones that cannot be seen or conveniently splinted, such as broken ribs, are usually not of immediate concern when offering first aid.

Burns → Cool (usually water)

Burns and scalds can range from very mild to life threatening and can affect any part of the body. Burns may be caused by intense heat (fire), solar radiation (sunburn) or chemicals (caustics/acids.) Since some form of heat generally causes burns, they usually feel hot. When things are too hot we instinctively want to cool them off. The conditioned response to burns is to cool them. The universal cooling agent is water.

If the area of a burn is fairly small and mobile, a hand or forearm for example, simply holding it under running tap water may be best. A larger area such as a chest or abdomen may be more easily treated in a cool shower or with a cool wet cloth. In nearly all instances, treating burns with a cool water rinse or cool wet towel is preferable.

Burns are generally more severe than they initially appear. Skin that is only slightly red at first may be blistered and oozing several hours later. For anything more than a very minor burn, you should assist the victim to get a medical evaluation as soon as possible.

Burns are extremely susceptible to infection. Try to keep burned areas clean, especially if the skin is broken. Use sterile dressings when available. If sterile dressings are not available, it's ok to gently cover the burn with a clean moist cloth (towel, clothing, etc.). It is acceptable to gently apply salves (bag balm, etc.) to very minor burns, but burns should never be rubbed with anything. The use of cool water to ease the burning sensation is the safest method.

Anyone who's experienced even a minor burn knows how extremely painful a burn can be. Burns should be handled gently, dressed lightly and evaluated by medical personnel as soon as possible.

A person who is overwhelmed by prolonged exposure to heat is said to have heat exhaustion or heat stroke if their mental status is affected. You should think of them as having a whole body "burn" and they can best be treated in the first aid setting by externally cooling with cool (not cold) water and encouraging them to drink generous amounts of cool liquids.

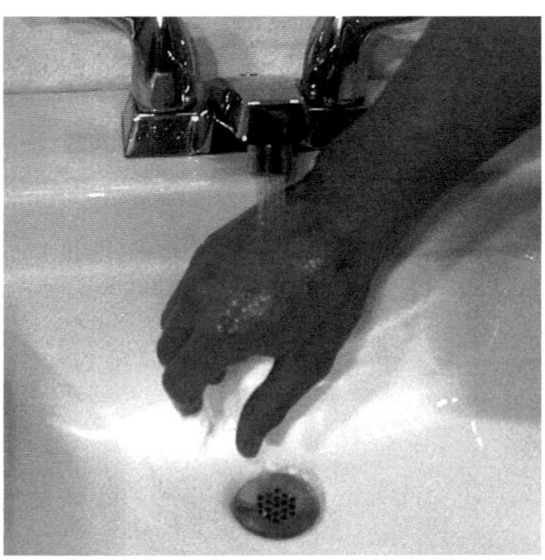

Cooling a burned hand under cool tap water

Bites ➔ Cover

There is an endless number of possible "bite" wounds. A partial list includes bites inflicted by teeth (animals, humans, etc.) bites (stings) from insects, coral or jellyfish, venomous bites from snakes and "bites" from extreme cold (frostbite). The condition-response for any bite is to cover the wound.

Although it may seem odd to include all of these injuries in the same Basic category, they actually have a lot in common. First, and most obviously, they are all commonly referred to as "bites". Second, although they seem different, they all respond to similar treatment: being "covered" in the emergency setting.

The following examples demonstrate the rationale for covering just about all of the injuries we call bites. When you cover an animal or human bites that have broken the skin you are able to provide pressure to help control bleeding and protecting the wound from further contamination. Bites (stings) from insects and aquatic life should be covered to provide comfort and minimize scratching and rubbing, which can increase sensitivity and invite infection. It is also reasonable to "cover" insect "bites" with ice to help control pain and itching.

Although frostbite is not really a bite wound, it has "bite" in its name and is best treated in the same manner as other "bites;" by wrapping (covering) the extremity to gradually re-warm it. Frostbite should not be treated with direct heat, nor should it be rubbed, since either action can damage frozen tissues.

Hypothermia may be viewed as a whole body frostbite that is treated by gradual re-warming to include covering the victim with a blanket.

There are countless salves, ointments, herbs, oils, foods, lotions, potions and creams that have been touted for the topical treatment of bite wounds. In general, first-aid rescuers shouldn't put anything in an open wound. On the other hand, it's usually harmless to put any of these products on a closed wound if it provides comfort to the victim.

Snakebite wounds should be covered while immediate medical help is sought. Since specific antivenom is often available, professional medical help should be obtained as soon as possible. You should not cut into snakebite wounds, try to "suck out the poison" or use tourniquets.

Baffled → Observe

The sixth B stands for baffled. The actual cause of a victim's distress may not be apparent. This is a common situation even for trained medical personnel. If you don't know what's wrong with a victim, you should continue to observe them while waiting for help. While you are observing them one of the first five Bs may become apparent and require the appropriate response. Sometimes the problem may appear to resolve entirely, but the person should still be observed because the problem can re-emerge without warning later. All but the most minor of baffling situations should be evaluated by trained medical personnel as soon as possible.

Specific Diagnoses

You may be concerned about being able to manage victims with specific diagnoses. There are, of course, hundreds of specific diagnoses and learning the specific response to each of them would be an overwhelming task. That's why Common Sense Lifesaving is condition centered instead of diagnosis centered. By experiencing the six Basics and their instinctive responses, you will be able to provide emergency assistance to the vast majority of emergency victims. Let's look at a couple of examples of broad diagnoses and how Common Sense Lifesaving will help you help these victims.

Management of Shock

"Shock" refers to several different medical diagnoses that result in the breakdown of the circulatory, respiratory and/or nervous system of a sick or injured person. Severe infection or exposure to toxins can cause shock. Heavy bleeding can cause shock from blood loss. Extreme heat or cold can overwhelm the body's ability to adapt and cause shock. Electrical and head injuries can also cause shock. It is unlikely that you would be able to recognize and apply definitive treatment for these many different kinds of shock, but, by applying CPR and the 6 Basics to the observed condition of a person who is suffering shock, the best possible first aid can be provided.

The problem of shock aptly demonstrates the importance of a simple, condition–response based approach to first aid for elementary providers. For example, in shock caused by bleeding – apply pressure. For shock due to head trauma, you should observe the victim closely and offer CPR and the 6 Basics as needed until medical help arrives.

Injuries Caused by Electricity

Another example of the application of Common Sense Lifesaving to a diagnostic group is electrical injuries. Electrocution is an electrical injury severe enough to compromise breathing or pulse, therefor CPR should be performed. Lesser electrical injuries that appear to cause superficial (skin) injury should be managed as Burns. Electrical injuries have the potential to cause internal damage and you should observe victims for the emergence of these problems at a later time. In general, nearly all electrical injuries should be referred for further medical care.

Automatic External Defibrillator (AED)

The automatic external defibrillator (AED) is a handbag sized computerized electrocardiogram (EKG) with a battery. The AED is capable of diagnosing ventricular fibrillation and automatically delivering a measured electrical shock to the victim's heart to restart a normal rhythm. The AED is becoming widely available in public places and can be utilized by just about anyone. If you encounter an unconscious person and have close access to an AED, you simply open the lid to the AED and follow the instructions. These are usually in the form of a step by step audio, but most units also have graphic instructions clearly printed on the unit.

Opening the outer case usually activates the unit and starts the instructions to:

1. Place the two adhesive pads on the victims bare chest at either end of the heart area (a graphic shows the correct placement).
2. Wait for the AED to advise you to stay clear from the patient while the AED delivers one or more electrical charges to restart the patients normal rhythm or that you should resume CPR as needed for the victim.

There are several brands and models available but all work similar to the two steps above and are very simple to operate. If possible, familiarize yourself with the operation of the AED you are likely to be using in an emergency. AEDs can save lives but they do not remove the need for CPR in a non-breathing victim.

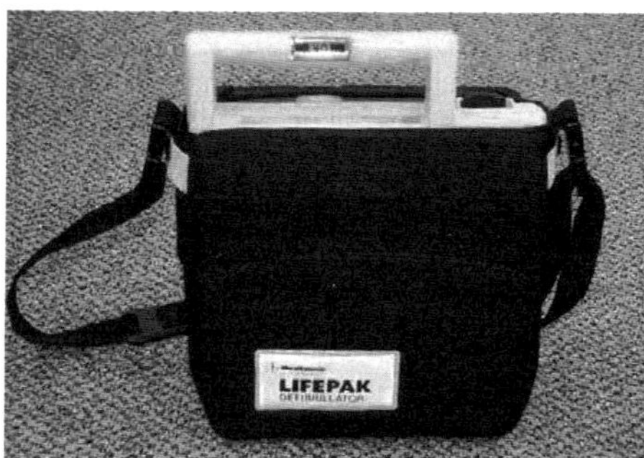

Automatic External Defibrillator (AED)

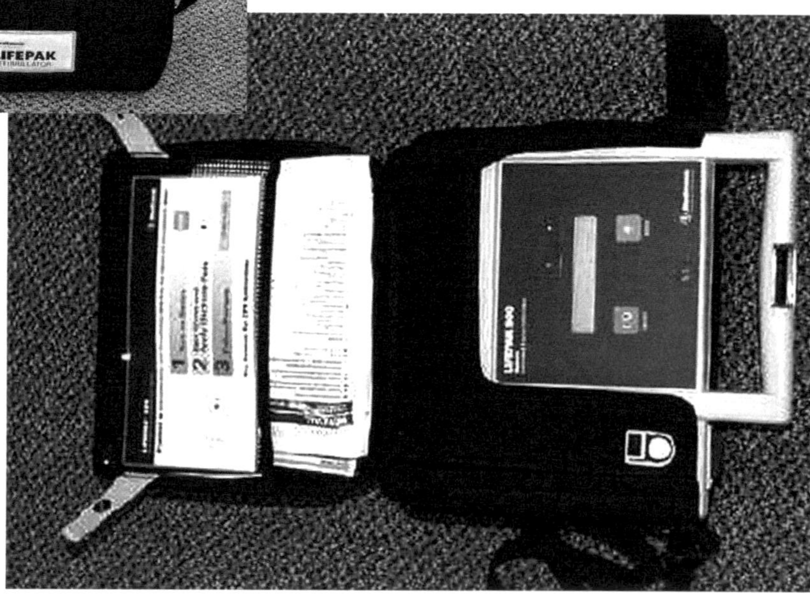

Giving Oxygen in an Emergency

"It is safe to give O2 to anyone who is badly injured."

Oxygen (O2) is the primary fuel for our bodies and giving O2 in an emergency helps assure that an injured or ill person has adequate energy to help them recover. There is no danger in giving O2 in the first aid setting.

The most intimidating thing about giving O2 for most rescuers is setting up and turning on unfamiliar equipment, especially since it is usually labeled with danger or warning stickers. Like most things, O2 can be dangerous if mishandled, but it is very safe to use O2 equipment as it was intended.

The cautions are simple; avoid extreme heat and don't directly expose pressurized O2 to flames, grease or oil.

O2 Equipment

Your choice of O2 supply will be dictated by what you have available. The non-rebreather mask is nearly universal.

Giving O2

There are only two steps to giving O2. The first step is to assemble (if needed) the regulator to the tank and turn on the O2. The second step is to connect the line and mask to the O2 supply and apply it to the victims face.

Oro-nasal mask with 02 inlet and one way valve

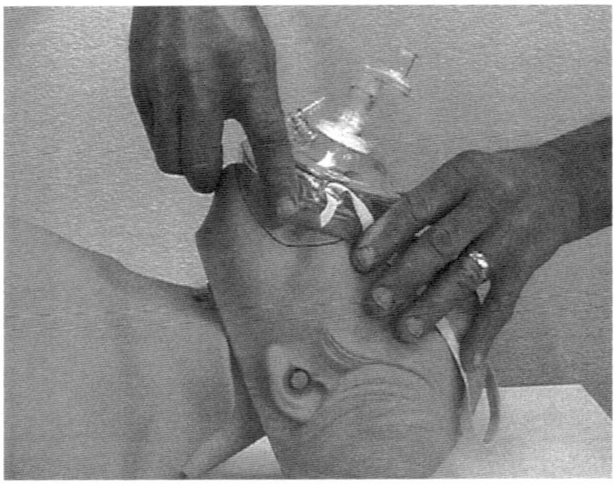

Non-rebreather mask on person's face-
Watch Airway!

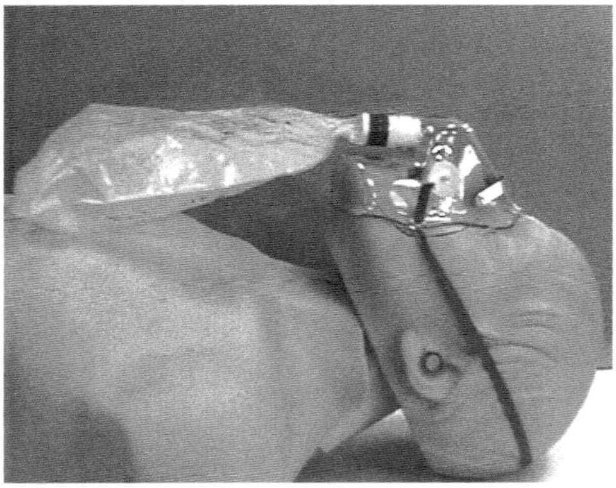

You use the key to turn on the bottle and select 15 LPM on the regulator. Then fit the mask snugly on the victims face. Note that the non-rebreather bag acts as a reservoir but need not fill between each breath. It is important to maintain airway and mask position in victims who are too weak to do so for themselves.

Practical O2

If possible, you should practice with the O2 equipment you are likely to have available in an emergency so you will be comfortable with it. Practice connecting the regulator to the valve, turning on the O2 and setting it to 15 liters per minute. Try fitting the mask to another person and to yourself. Be sure you experience breathing O2 through the mask to increase your comfort level with its use.

CPR - The response to not breathing

CPR is the most dramatic and intimidating of all first-aid procedures. CPR is also the most important first-aid response and should always be given first if needed. Common Sense Lifesaving is structured to make the skill of CPR more "approachable" by eliminating anatomy and physiology and by utilizing the "Rule of 2s" to make CPR simpler and easier to remember.

Almost half of the people in America die of heart attack and many of those lives could be saved by CPR. Unfortunately, only a small percent of the public is CPR trained. There are many reasons for this disappointing statistic but one problem is that CPR & first-aid training are perceived as time consuming, expensive & confusing. Sadly, even those who are trained often fail to offer help in an emergency. Reasons for this failure to act include "I forgot what to do" and "I was afraid I would hurt the victim."

Many emergency professionals have concluded that CPR must become simpler to learn, easier to remember and less intimidating to use in an emergency. Common Sense Lifesaving has been designed from the ground up to accomplish the goals of CPR with AED, O2 administration and first-aid.

CPR is the process by which a person (rescuer) mechanically the delivers of O_2 to the lungs and circulation of blood throughout the body of another person (victim) whose heart or breathing has failed. You only need to know a few simple concepts to effectively provide CPR.

The human body requires oxygen to function. We inhale O_2 (in air) into our lungs where it is absorbed by our blood and carried to our brain, body organs and other tissues. The flow of blood through heart, lungs and body tissues and back again is called circulation. Our heart is the pump that circulates the blood.

Breathing in delivers fresh O_2 to our lungs to be absorbed by the circulating blood and breathing out gets rid of the stale CO_2 from our circulating blood. The process is very simple; inhale O_2 - circulate it through our body - exhale bad CO_2, over and over again in a continuous lifelong cycle.

Failure of either process, breathing or circulation, results in inadequate O_2 delivery to the tissues and the tissues will become damaged or die. Lack of fresh O_2 causes injury to the heart and brain within seconds. We call injury to these organs heart attack or stroke, respectively. Damage to either organ can be fatal.

CPR can be lifesaving and the Rule of 2s was developed to help you learn and remember the essential steps of CPR.

CPR *(refer to CPR side of your slate)*

As you approach the scene of what appears to be an emergency with a victim:

- **Assess Scene and Person Involved in Incident**

  Assess scene & victim: Assess the situation, consider both the victim and surroundings. The excitement of an actual rescue scenario and the desire to help others can result in an impulsive rescue attempt. Approaching an unsafe scene can lead to you becoming a victim (smoke, electrical, traffic, etc.). Also, protect yourself by donning protective clothing (gloves, masks, etc.) if available and appropriate.

- **Alert EMS**

  Alert the emergency medical system: You should do this for almost any accident or emergency, especially if there are injuries and always if there is any doubt. The timing for alerting EMS varies and will depend on circumstances such as other rescuers, communications and the urgency of the situation.

- **Approach Person. Statement "Are you OK?"**

  Approach a possible victim and determine if CPR is required "Are you OK?" "I can help". Many people are shy about coming forward in an emergency. The exact words they use are less important than just saying something. Try talking to the victim – if the victim can answer rationally they do not need CPR. Apply the 6 Basics and offer the victim O2 if available.

- **Person Breathing?**

  YES: Administer first aid follow steps on back of slate

  Normal breathing: Breathing can be assessed by listening and watching the chest for movement. A pulse can be difficult to locate in an emergency but breathing victims will almost always have a pulse. Breathing should be steady, not erratic or labored, to be satisfactory. If the victim is breathing effectively, CPR is not needed at the time, but you should reassess frequently.

  NO: Administer CPR

  If the victim's breathing is absent or not clearly detectable you need to breathe for the victim. Pulse may or may not be present, but attempting to verify a pulse is often difficult and can waste valuable time. It is safer to assume there is no pulse and provide CPR. As you move to provide CPR, you should ask other rescuers or bystanders to obtain an automatic external defibrillator (AED) if possible. A single rescuer should never delay or abandon CPR for more than a few seconds to seek an AED or other equipment. If an AED is available, CPR should be started and continued while a second rescuer retrieves and activates it. Once the AED is connected, follow its instructions but continue CPR as soon as it declines shock or completes it's shock sequence without restoring normal pulse and breathing.

ABCs -Airway, Breathing and Circulation

Effective CPR requires immediate placement of the victim on their back. This position is important for both maintaining the airway and giving effective compressions. Moving an injured victim onto their back does carry the remote risk of spinal cord damage in the event of a broken neck. Since victims may be encountered in an endless variety of positions there is no single maneuver for safely placing a victim on his/her back.

The main consideration is to stabilize the victims head in relationship to their shoulders. This is much simpler with two rescuers. You should practice rolling a limp 'victim' to get an idea of how to best stabilize their neck during movement.

> *"Never allow a victim to die from lack of CPR because of the remote possibility of spinal cord injury."*

Open Airway: The A in the ABCs.

One of the most important components in successful CPR is getting the victims head into the correct position help keep the breathing path from mouth to lungs (the airway) open. You should practice using the head tilt, chin lift method. If rescue breaths will not go in, gently reposition the head and try again. If breaths still will not go in, an obstruction may be present. Perform a finger sweep of the mouth to check for obstructions. The most common airway obstruction is the victim's own tongue and throat structures, but obstructions may also include vomitus, dentures, gum or chewing tobacco. A finger sweep is usually effective in clearing the blockage. If you get the head position right, the airway and breathing portion of CPR will probably go very smoothly.

Be gentle but positive in obtaining a good airway. There is a tiny risk of spinal cord damage if the victim's neck is broken but a victim who is not breathing will surely die if you do not obtain an airway!

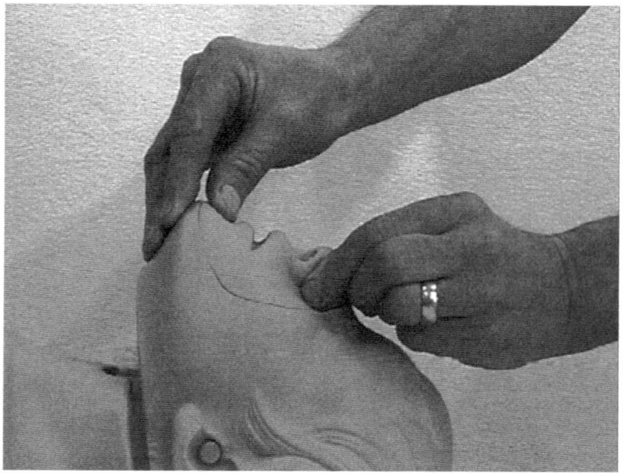

- **Provide Breathing and Circulation**

  (*Refer to the steps on your slate to provide breathing and circulation*)

- **Chin Lift and Gentle Head Tilt - Protect Neck!**

Follow Rule of 2s

The Rule of 2s is a memory device to help you remember the practical dimensions of CPR and O2 delivery. It simplifies all the numbers to remember to the number 2 with 2 exceptions, which are 15 for O2 and 30 for compressions.

Give 2 Full Breaths - Blow in for 2 Seconds Each

Pinch or cover the victim's nose (with an oro-nasal mask) and breathe into mouth or mask inlet. Give 2 full breaths (each about 2 seconds long) to make the victims chest rise and fall. Use the oro-nasal mask when it is available. Be sure to maintain good victim neck/jaw position while giving rescue breaths. You should practice both with and without the oro-nasal mask.

You will be blowing air into the victim's lungs for him. Just blow right into his/her mouth, either directly or through the oro-nasal mask if available. Remember to block the victim's nose so your breath doesn't leak right back out. You can tell if it's working by watching their chest rise and fall.

Stack 2 Hands 2 Fingers up from Bottom of Sternum

Position your upper body directly above and perpendicular to your victim's chest. Place the palm of one hand over the victim's breastbone and stack your other hand on top of your own hand. Your arms should be extended almost straight and vertically down to the victim's chest. This position will let you use your own body weight to assist in chest compressions and will help you avoid tiring quickly.

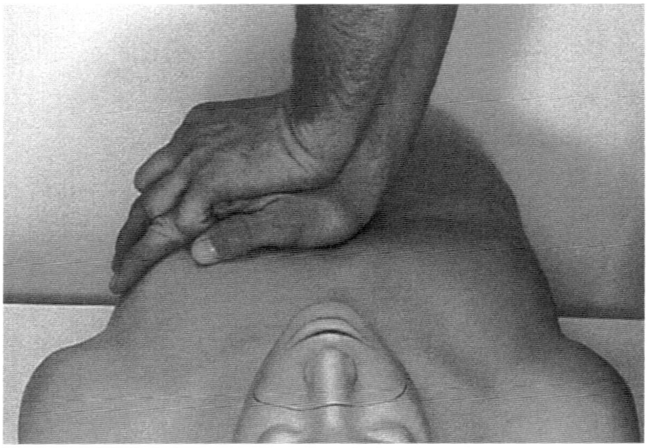

Compress 2" (about 2 fat fingers) less than 2x a second

The recommended depth of compression is 1-2 inches. Do not be too cautious about chest compression out of fear that you will "hurt" the victim. Inadequate compressions fail to restore circulation and can contribute to the victim's death, while compressing more than necessary may cause chest wall injury but still sustain life. Err on the side of generous compressions. The recommended rate of compressions is 80 to 100 per minute. Timing compressions is difficult at best, especially for a lone rescuer. Applying compressions a little slower than 2 compressions per second results in a fair approximation of the ideal rate.

Two Exceptions

Now it's time to introduce the 2 exceptions. Most rules have exceptions. The Rule of 2s has 2 exceptions.

1st Exception:

- **After 30 compressions - repeat breath cycle**. A lone rescuer should give 30 compressions between every two breaths.
- **Two rescuers breath two times as often.**

  If there are two rescuers, one rescuer should give two breaths after the other rescuer gives 15 compressions. Accurate counting is not as important as establishing a fluid and rhythmic pattern. Do not be concerned if you lose count and provide a few more or less than 30 (15 for two rescuers) compressions between breath cycles. The most important factor is that you are providing CPR at all. Just continue and do your best.
- **Apply AED (if available) after two cycles**

  If an AED is available, it may be applied after two cycles. You need to open and activate the unit and follow its audio instructions. In the case of a lone rescuer, this will interrupt CPR. The rescuer should never allow a non-breathing victim to go without CPR for more than two minutes.
- **Reassess periodically but continue CPR as long as needed**

2nd Exception:

Give O2 @ 15 lpm if available - requires oro-nasal mask

- If O2 is available and can be connected to an oro-nasal mask without delaying CPR for more than a few seconds, set O2 flow rate at 15 LPM and give 2 rescue breaths through the tube on top of the mask every 15 compressions just as you would in CPR without O2. It is vital that you do not compromise their CPR efforts to connect O2.

"Be Persistent - You're Saving a Life!"

Continue as long as necessary or until EMS arrives. Remember that even if their efforts are less than "textbook", you may be giving the victim the only chance he has. Any effort at all is heroic.

Rescue and Transport of Casualties

The practical aspects of physical rescue and transport of casualties is as variable as first aid itself. Assess the scene and approach with caution. Alert EMS (call for help) as soon as possible. Provide CPR and first aid to victim(s) being mindful of potential hazards to yourself and other rescuers. Avoid harming victims further (ex. unnecessary movement of the neck) but, do not withhold CPR or needed first aid out of fear of harming the victim.

Transportation for medical help for victims who need it should be arranged as soon as possible. Emergency transport may be by boat, air, ground ambulance or private vehicle as deemed appropriate to the situation. Generally, the most important criteria for selecting transport is safety for rescuer and victim. Transportation under emergency conditions can become a hazard in itself. It is often best to wait for the arrival of trained emergency personnel for safe transport. Remember, needed CPR and first aid must be continued during transportation of victims

Talk Calmly, Offer Comfort, Don't Force

Being calm in an emergency can be one of a rescuer's most important tools. It helps to defuse the panic and confusion that is often present. Your calmness instills confidence and puts victim(s) and other rescuers at ease. Calmness promotes clear thinking and useful responses.

Providing comfort is one of the most instinctive and human of all responses. Nearly all people respond positively to physical and emotional comfort and it can give measurable benefit. In many situations, providing reassurance and comfort may be the most significant thing you can offer.

In keeping with a positive and supportive approach to victims of accident or illness, remember that victims still have legal rights. Although certified paramedics have limited police powers while on duty, first-aid providers do not. A victim of an accident or illness may for whatever reason, refuse a rescuer's assistance. The injured individual has the right to refuse emergency care unless it directly and immediately endangers him or others. Repeated attempts to force a victim to accept treatment will often cause the victim to refuse all help and can occasionally create hazards for those involved. By demonstrating your respect for a victim's rights, you are more likely to be trusted and can more effectively render assistance.

Common Questions About Lifesaving

Bleeding

Can I get a disease such as AIDS from contact with a victim's blood?

Yes, but it is unlikely. First, the victim must have the disease. Secondly, the blood must enter your circulation through a break in the skin's protective barrier. Such transmission is extremely rare in the first-aid scenario, but it does provide good reason for being cautious and avoiding unnecessary contact with a victim's body fluids. Be sure to wash thoroughly after contact with anyone, but do not be afraid to help a victim!

Why aren't we taught to use pressure points?

Pressure points require knowledge of circulatory anatomy and can be difficult to find even for a trained medical professional. You should not attempt to add this complexity and confusion to the simple and rememberable format of CPROX1st.

How are nosebleeds treated?

Bleeding - Pressure. You need to have the victim squeeze their nose to apply pressure to the inside of the nose. If the bleed persists, they should seek medical help.

Why don't we use tourniquets?

Tourniquets cut off the blood supply to everything beyond them, not just the wound, and can cause serious tissue damage. Direct pressure slows the blood from leaking out of the wound and is the correct method.

CPR

Can I hurt the victim by moving their head for CPR?

There is a slight chance of damaging the spinal cord by moving the head if there has been serious head-neck trauma. However, if a victim is not breathing and needs CPR, they are likely to die quickly without effective ventilation. Therefore, the risk is a slight chance of paralysis versus a high likelihood of death. The answer is to position the victim's head as carefully as possible - especially if there is evidence of head-neck trauma - but effective rescue breathing is the absolute priority.

Why was the recommended number of compressions changed from 15 to 30?

There is evidence that compressions alone are helpful in ventilation. Frequent position changes every 15 compressions are complicated and tiring for a single rescuer. For two trained rescuers, the recommendation remains at 15 compressions each cycle. This is confusing to non-professionals and therefore CPROX1st teaches 30 compressions per cycle for general rescue purposes.

What if I can't get rescue breaths through the victim's mouth?

Try to clear any obstructions from the victim's mouth using a sweep of your finger. It's OK to try several times but don't waste more than a few seconds before trying an alternate route such as their nose.

What if I want to help but I don't want to put my mouth on the victims?

It is desirable to use a barrier of some kind. It can be a commercial device or as simple as a layer of clothing such as a shirt. If you are absolutely unwilling or unable to give rescue breathes, perform chest compressions anyway as chest compressions alone have been shown to be useful.

Diabetes

What is diabetes?

Diabetes is a medical condition that can result in a victim having too much or too little sugar in their blood. A first-aid provider cannot differentiate between the two situations. Giving sugar containing foods or drinks can correct low blood sugar and is not likely to make high blood sugar significantly worse. Therefore, if there is doubt, offer a diabetic victim something sweet. Do not force them. Don't try to give sweet food or drink to an unconscious victim as it may cause them to aspirate and choke. Follow the Basics.

Heart Attack

How do I tell if a person is having a heart attack?

A heart attack can present with or without chest pain, shortness of breath, sweating or nausea. Heart attack often mimics indigestion. First-aid givers cannot accurately diagnose heart problems. If heart trouble is suspected, get help. Follow the Basics.

Poisoning

How do I help a person who has been poisoned?

Try to determine what they may have been poisoned by. Call 911 and request the poison control center. Follow the Basics.

Pulse

Why don't we emphasize checking a victim's pulse in CPR?

Finding a victim's pulse can be very difficult even under ideal circumstances. Searching for a pulse in an emergency can waste critical moments. Even if a pulse is felt it may be 1) sub-optimal for resuscitation or 2) the rescuers own pulse. A regular pattern of breathing strongly suggests a pulse is also present and if a victim is not breathing, time should not be wasted trying to evaluate the pulse. It is safest to provide full CPR.

Seizures

How do I help a person having a seizure?

Seizures may be focal or generalized (grand mal). Generalized seizures involve the entire body and may last for several minutes. The purpose of first-aid in a generalized seizure is to help prevent the victim from injuring himself during or after the seizure. Try to provide comfort. Do not attempt to put anything in the mouth of a seizing person. Follow the Basics.

Shock

What is shock?

Shock is a critical lack of oxygen being circulated to the brain and vital organs.

What causes shock?

There are many causes of shock such as bleeding, heart attack or massive internal injuries. They can be difficult to diagnose even in the medical setting. This is a major reason why it is important for you to focus on the Basics as the best response to shock.

Is fainting the same as shock?

Simple fainting is a minor and very transient form of shock that is self-correcting. It may be associated with an emotional reaction. Even though fainting generally resolves without harm, it should always be followed up with a medical evaluation.

Stroke

What is a stroke?

A stroke is usually a sudden loss of oxygen to a portion of the brain. When this happens, that part of the brain is injured or dies and the part of the body controlled by that part of the brain is paralyzed, for example, speech or one side of the body. Strokes can be very small or massive. Although strokes may improve in the days that follow, they may be permanent or even become worse. Follow the Basics.

Notes:

Notes: